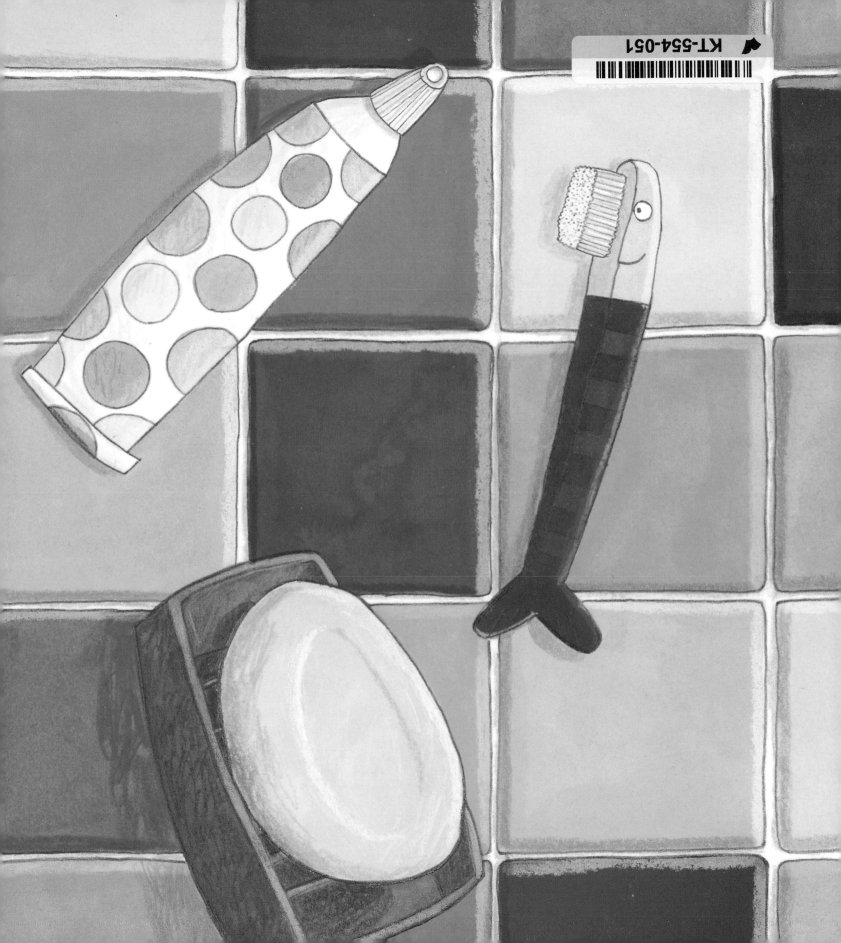

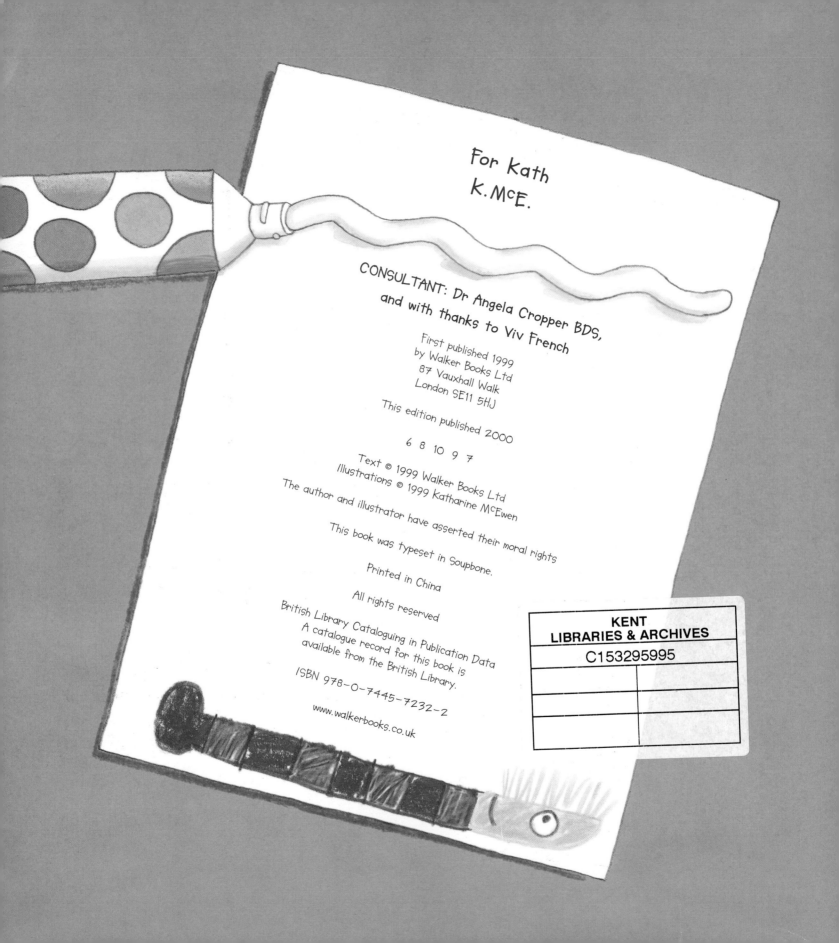

For Kath
K. McE.

CONSULTANT: Dr Angela Cropper BDS,
and with thanks to Viv French

First published 1999
by Walker Books Ltd
87 Vauxhall Walk
London SE11 5HJ

This edition published 2000

6 8 10 9 7

This book was typeset in Soupbone.

Printed in China

British Library Cataloguing in Publication Data
A catalogue record for this book is
available from the British Library.

ISBN 978-0-7445-7232-2

www.walkerbooks.co.uk

I KNOW WHY I BRUSH MY TEETH

KATE ROWAN

illustrated by

KATHARINE McEWEN

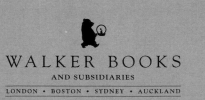

WALKER BOOKS
AND SUBSIDIARIES

LONDON · BOSTON · SYDNEY · AUCKLAND

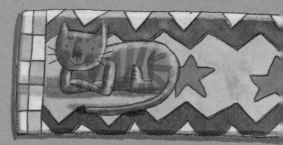

"MUM!"
yelled Sam.
"Come here, QUICK!"

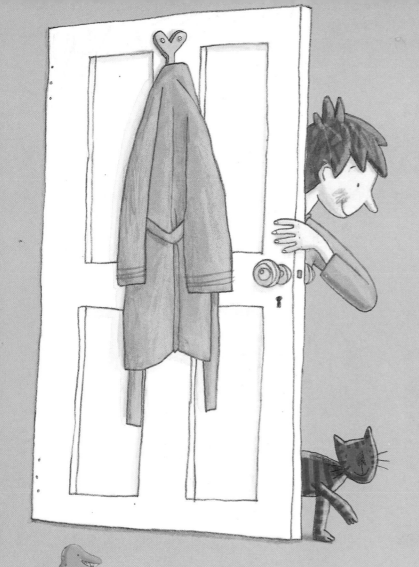

"What is it, Sam?"
asked Mum.
"Aren't you ready
for your bath yet?"

"LOOK!" said Sam proudly.
"I've got a wobbly
tooth!"

"Hmm," said Mum,
peering into
his mouth,
"so you have."

big tooth

baby tooth

gum

JAW BONE

"That means it's
going to fall out,
doesn't it?" said Sam.
"A big tooth is starting
to push the baby tooth
out of the way — that's
what the dentist said."

"That's right," Mum said, passing Sam his toothbrush and toothpaste, "but not for a few days yet. Come on, let's give those teeth a really good clean."

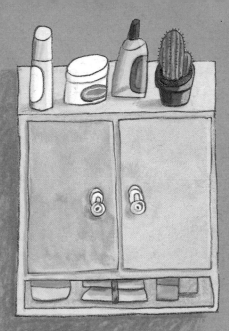

Mum frowned.

"SAM! That's FAR
too much toothpaste!
Remember what else
the dentist said."

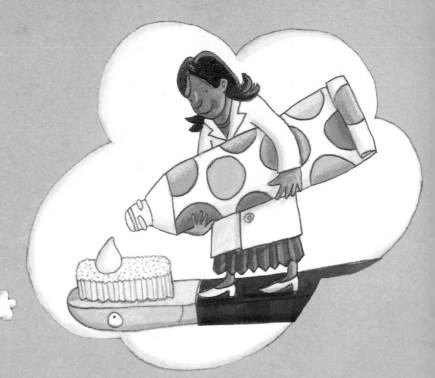

"I know, I know," said Sam.
"Only use a pea-sized blob
of toothpaste, 'cos it's
got floor stuff in it,
and I only need
a little bit of
the floor stuff."

"You mean **fluoride**," said Mum.

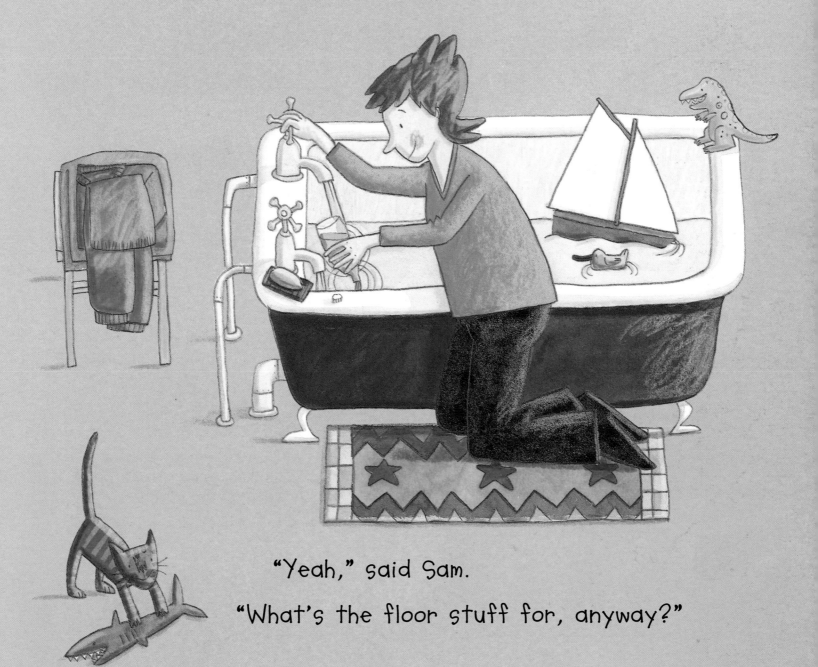

"Yeah," said Sam.

"What's the floor stuff for, anyway?"

"It helps to keep your teeth strong," explained Mum.

11

"I'VE got strong teeth," Sam said.
"AND I haven't got any holes.
Jody in my class has holes.
Her mum says it's 'cos she eats
too many sweets."

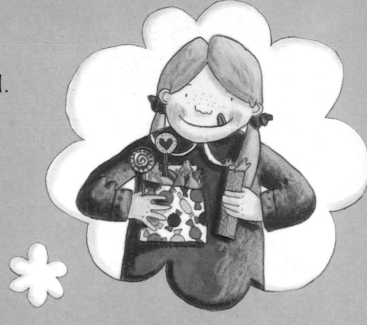

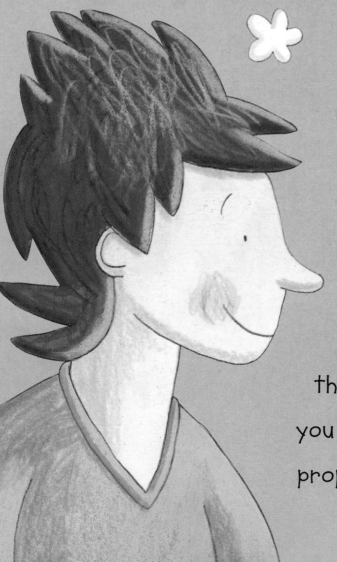

"I expect it is,"
said Mum. "Poor Jody.
It's not just sweets that
can give you holes, though.
Sugary drinks and snacks
between meals aren't good
for your teeth either,
especially if you don't clean
them often enough. That's why
you should brush your teeth
properly, at least twice a day."

"I know how to do it properly," Sam said. "The dentist showed me. Open wide and scrub backwards and forwards along the tops and insides. Then teeth together and round and round on the outsides. Look, I'll show you."

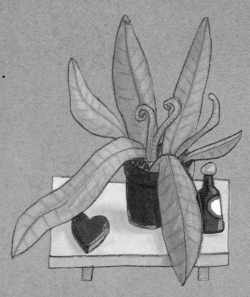

"That's great!" said Mum. "Don't forget to rinse your mouth out with clean water when you're done."

Sam peered at his
teeth in the mirror.
"Why does brushing
stop the holes?"

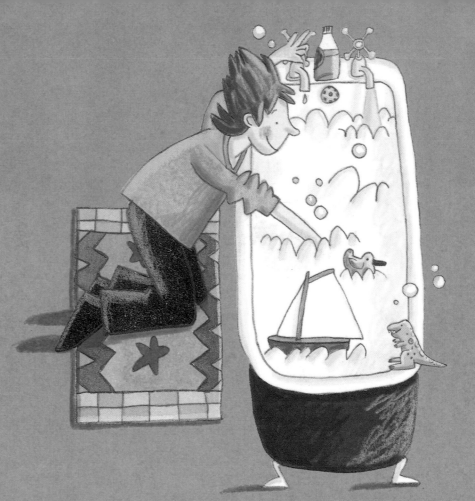

"It's because little bits
of food stick to your teeth
when you eat," said Mum.
"If you don't brush them away,
germs called **bacteria** get to work
on them and form gooey stuff
that builds up on your teeth.

"The gooey stuff's called **plaque**," explained Mum,
"and the **bacteria** in the **plaque** feed on the sugar
in the food bits. This makes a very strong liquid
called **acid**, which eats into the outside of
your teeth and makes holes in them."

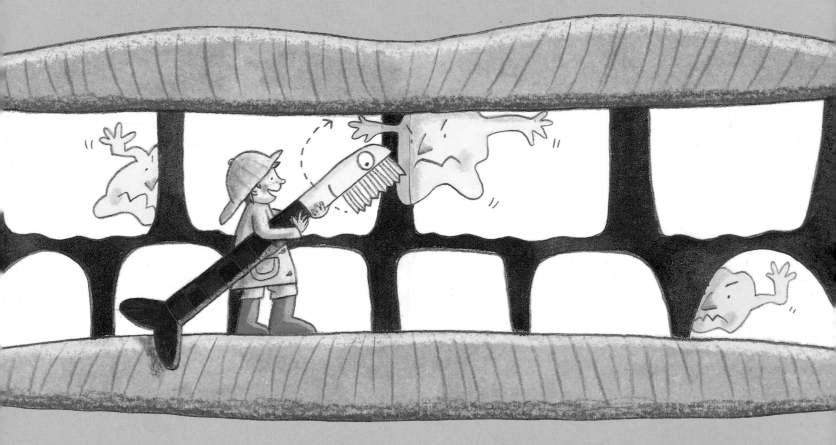

"Oh," said Sam, as he climbed into the bath.
"Do teeth have an outside and an inside then?"

"Yes they do," said Mum. "The shiny white stuff on the outside is called **enamel**, and it's really hard, like armour. In fact, **enamel** is the hardest thing in your whole body!"

"What's more," she added, "underneath the enamel there's bony stuff called **dentine**, and inside that there's **pulp**. **Pulp** is soft and squishy, and it's got lots of tiny **blood vessels** and things called **nerves** in it."

16

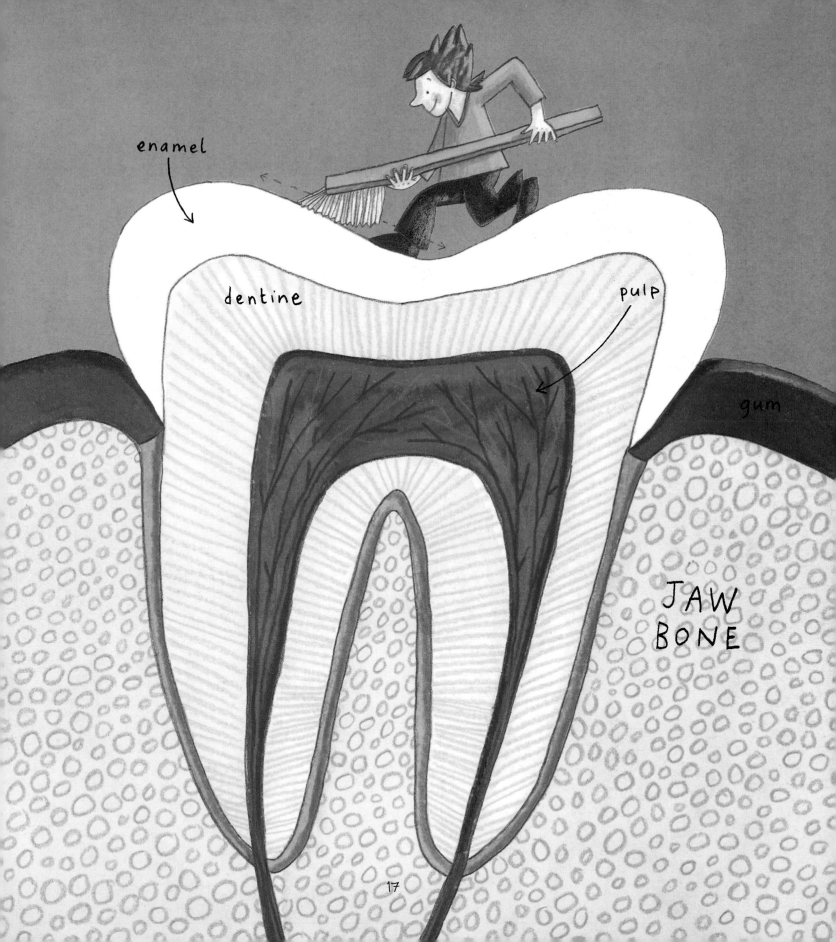

enamel

dentine

pulp

gum

JAW
BONE

17

"I know about **nerves**," Sam said.
"When I touch something, they tell
me if it's hot or cold.

"That's one of the things they do,"
said Mum. "**Nerves** tell you when
something's hurting you, too —
like that time I had a hole
in one of my teeth and
I got toothache."

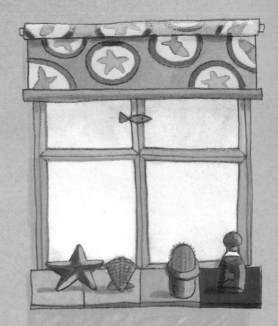

18

Sam made a face. "Yuck! I hope I never get toothache."

Mum smiled. "I hope you don't either, but that's why it's so important to take care of your teeth. You'll only grow one set of big teeth, and they'll have to last you the rest of your life."

"Will ALL my baby teeth fall out now?" asked Sam.

"They will," said Mum, "but not all at once. You've got twenty baby teeth altogether, and they'll come out one at a time over the next few years."

"I know why they're called baby teeth," Sam said. "It's because they started growing when I was a baby. But I'm not a baby anymore, am I? That's why I'm getting my big teeth!"

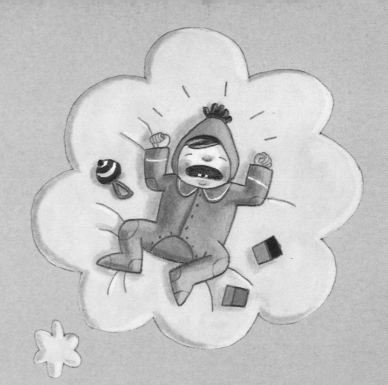

"That's right," said Mum. "You'll get thirty-two big teeth, and you'll have most of them by the time you're thirteen. But you won't get the very last ones, your **wisdom teeth**, until you're quite a bit older."

Sam nodded. "When I'm all grown up, you mean.

"Why are they called wisdom teeth?" Sam asked.

"Because you'll be older and wiser by the time you get them!" said Mum. "Your other teeth have names, too, you know."

"Do they?" asked Sam. "Like what?"

4 incisors in the middle, top and bottom

"Well, the teeth at the front are your **incisors**," said Mum. "They work like scissors to cut your food up. And the pointy ones next to them are the **canines**, or dog teeth. They're good for tearing and biting. Then the flat ones at the back are the **molars**. You use those for chewing and grinding up your food."

2 molars on each side, top and bottom

1 canine on each side, top and bottom

8 incisors + **8** molars + **4** canines = **20** baby teeth

Sam put on his pyjamas.
"Are the dog teeth
called that because
dogs have them, too?"

"I think they must be," Mum said.
"**Canine** is just another
way of saying dog."

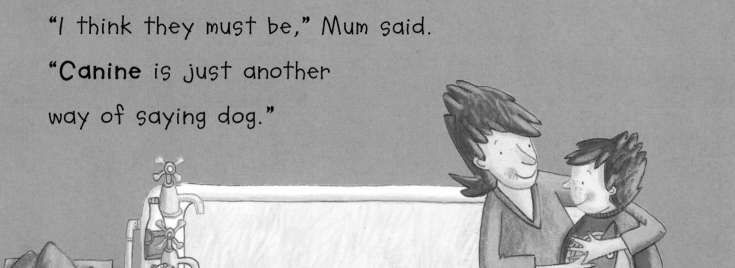

"Oh," said Sam. "Well I know an animal
that's got hundreds of teeth."

Mum laughed. "Oh do you?
What is it then?"

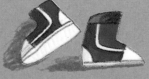

25

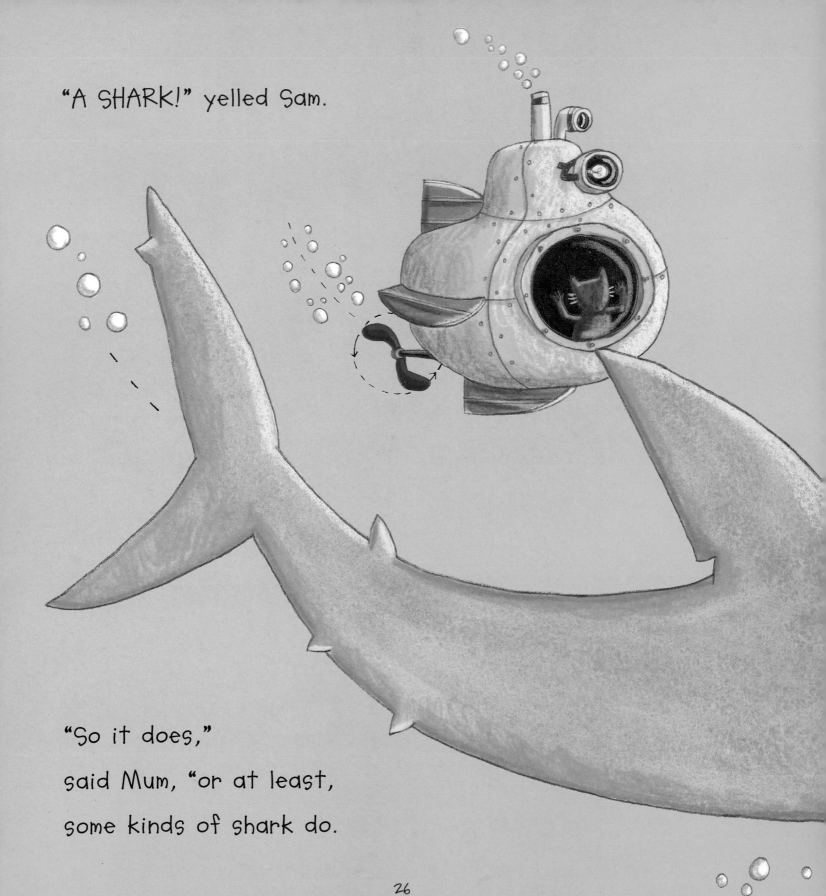

"A SHARK!" yelled Sam.

"So it does,"
said Mum, "or at least,
some kinds of shark do.

"And guess what," Mum went on.
"They're always losing their teeth
when they chomp on their food,
but they keep on growing
new ones all through
their lives."

"Well I'm not going
to lose any of my big
teeth when I get them,"
Sam said firmly.

"Good!" said Mum.

"Then you'll grow up to have beautiful big strong ones."

Sam grinned.

"All the better to eat you with..."

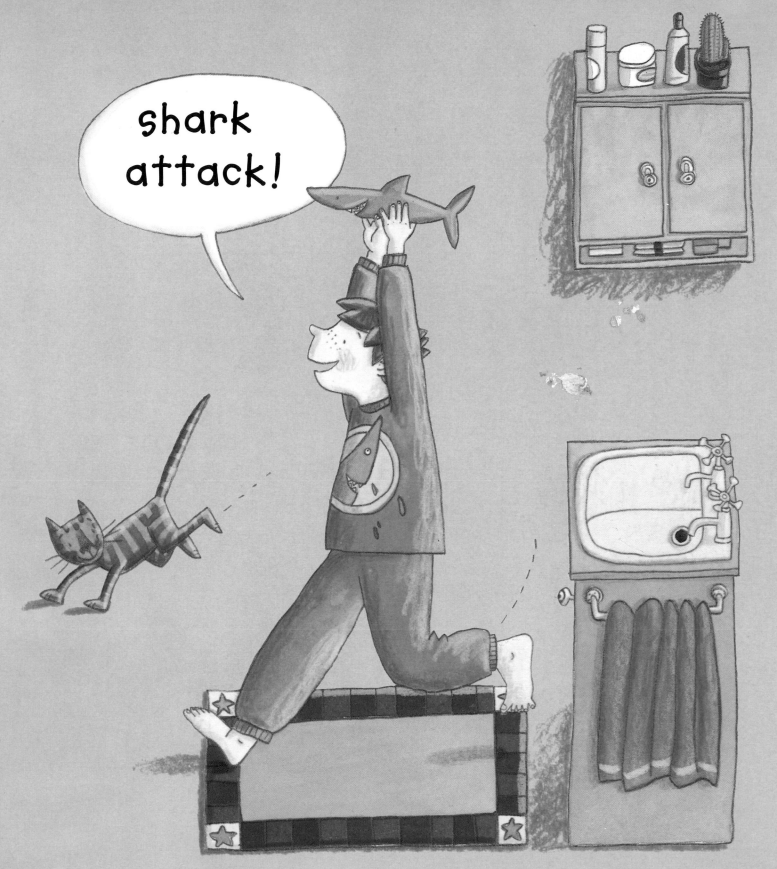

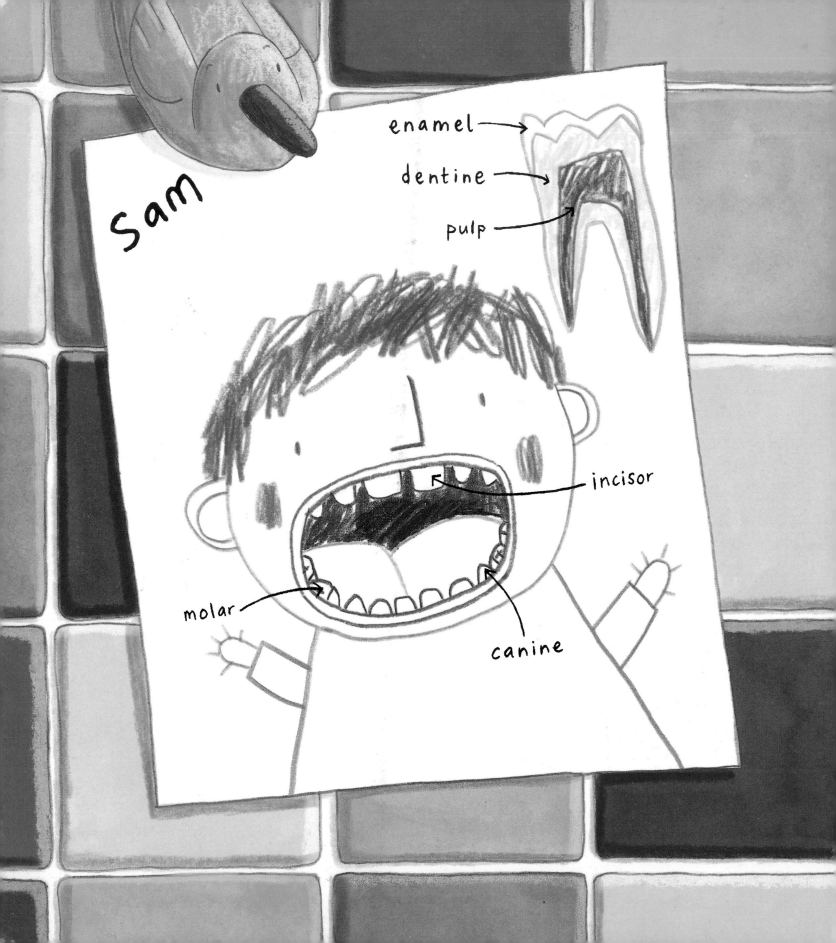

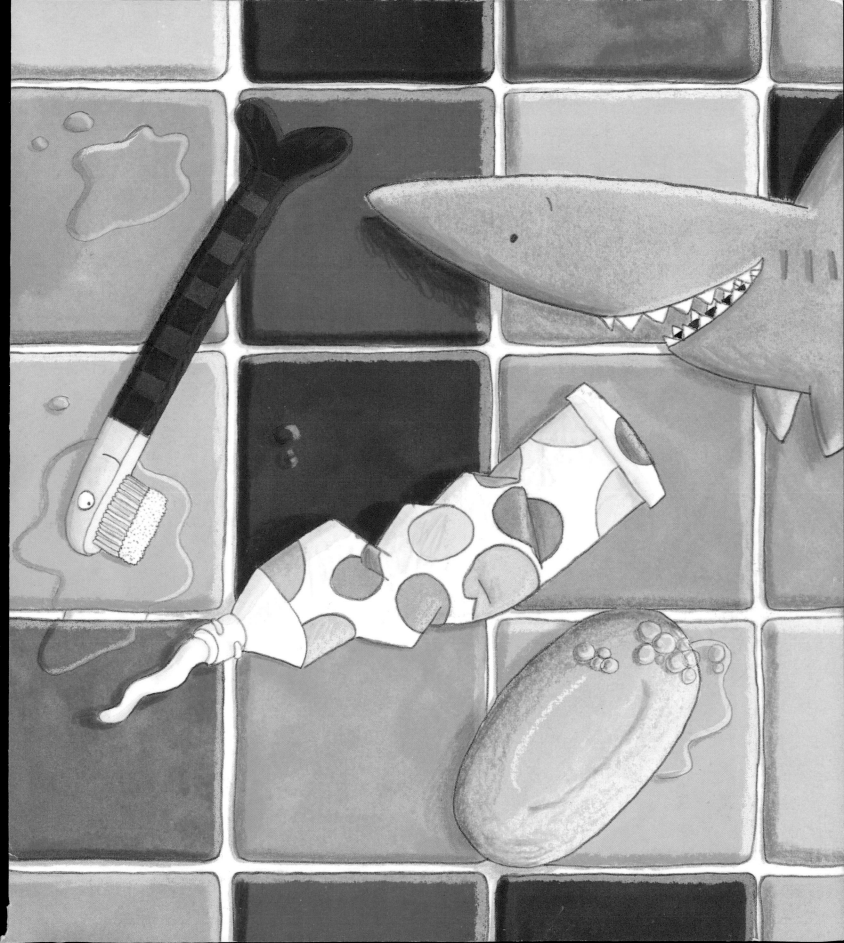

Index

Look up the pages to find out about all these teeth things.